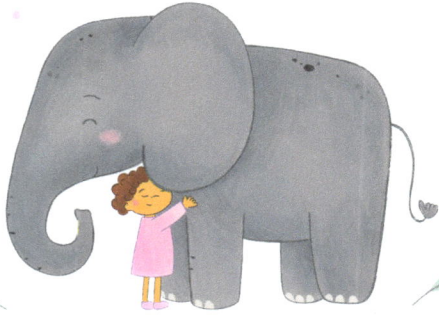

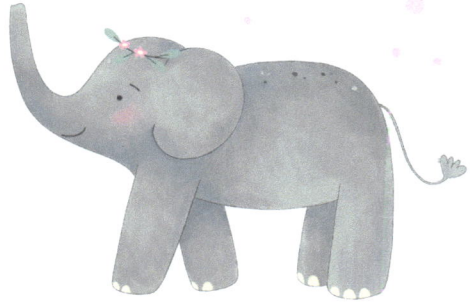

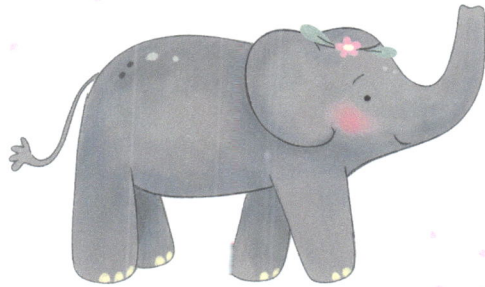

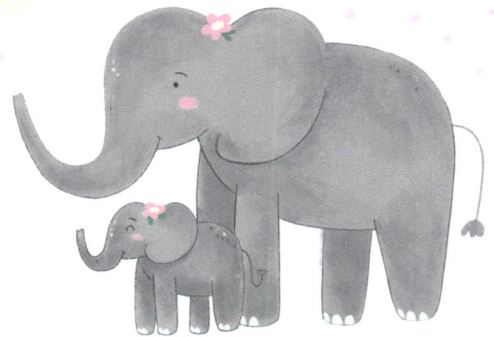

This book is dedicated to my 🩷 Elephant Bubbas 🩷

Independently published by
Play & Filial Therapy Press (Dr. Kate Renshaw)
www.drplay.com.au

First published by Dr. Kate Renshaw 2025©
Text copyright ©2025 Dr. Kate Renshaw
Illustrations copyright ©2025

For more information address Dr. Kate Renshaw
drkaterenshaw@gmail.com

A catalogue for this book is available at
the National Library of Australia

ISBN: 978-0-6458952-3-0

The artwork in this book is digitally created using Adobe Photoshop
Printed by Ingram Spark.

Hello Elephant Mumma!

Elephant Mumma, as you read aloud these words you are also reading to your Elephant Bubba.

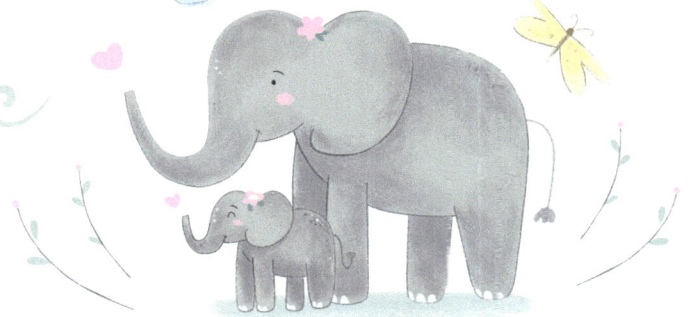

Written by Dr. Kate Renshaw

Illustrated by Roksolana Panchyshyn

Why elephants?

Elephants and humans share highly developed brain architecture and require the same ideal conditions for growth and development: sensitive, close, social attachment relationships.

With the longest pregnancy of all land-dwelling mammals, elephants practice patience and great strength, both physically and mentally, as they carry their unborn calf for close to two years. When humans studied traumatised elephants, they uncovered the wisdom of elephant parenting practices that include:

1. Strong emotional bonds and sense of attachment
2. Protective yet encouraging independence
3. Community and extended support networks
4. Patient, long-term nurturing

5. Teaching through modelling and gentle guidance

6. Unconditional love with clear boundaries

7. Emotional intelligence and communication

Elephants and humans both share highly developed brain architecture. We have more in common with elephants than you may realise, and elephant wisdom can help us better understand our own parenting. Share in both human and elephant wisdom as you become an Elephant Mumma to your Elephant Bubba.

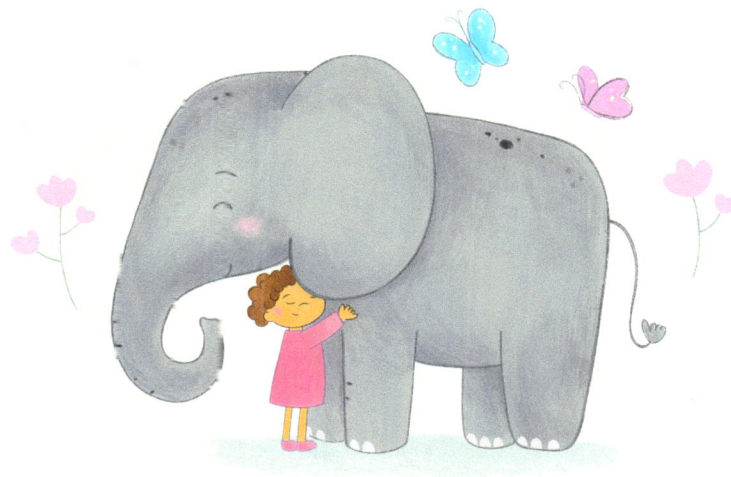

Before we get started, a note for Elephant Mummas.
As you carry your growing Elephant Bubba know that:

1. Your words are powerful
2. Your thoughts are powerful
3. Your feelings are powerful
4. And, your hopes are powerful too

P.S. The same goes for you Elephant Pappas.
And you can read this book aloud too!

"My words are powerful!"

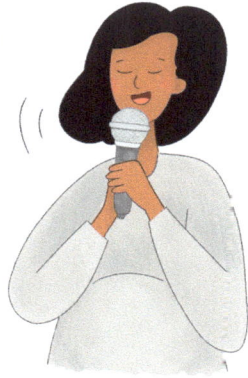

"My thoughts are powerful!"

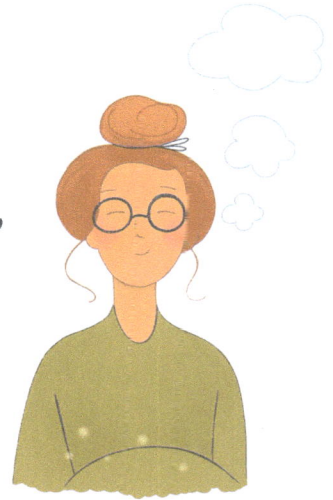

"My feelings are powerful!"

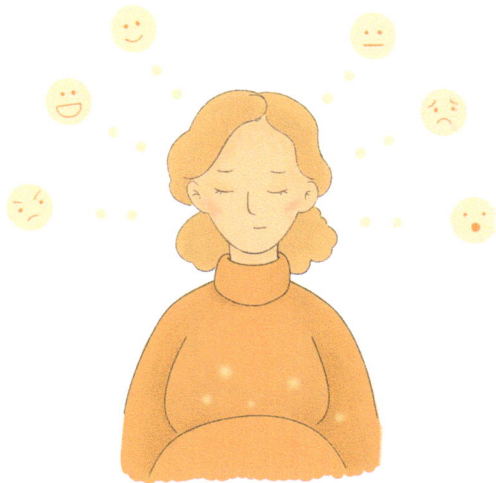

"My hopes are powerful too!"

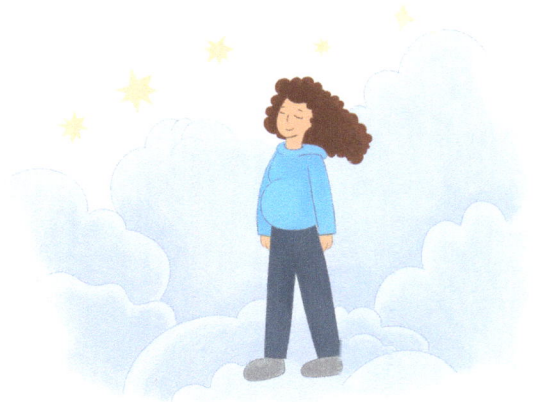

You are starting your journey Elephant Mumma!

Don't worry, I am here with you.

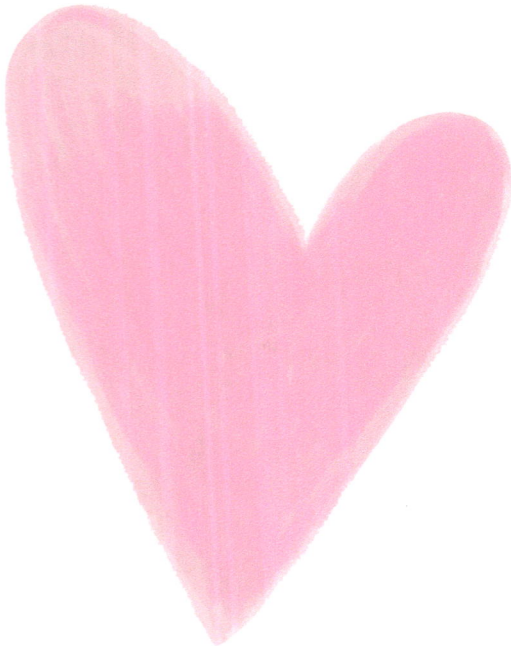

Elephant Bubba X

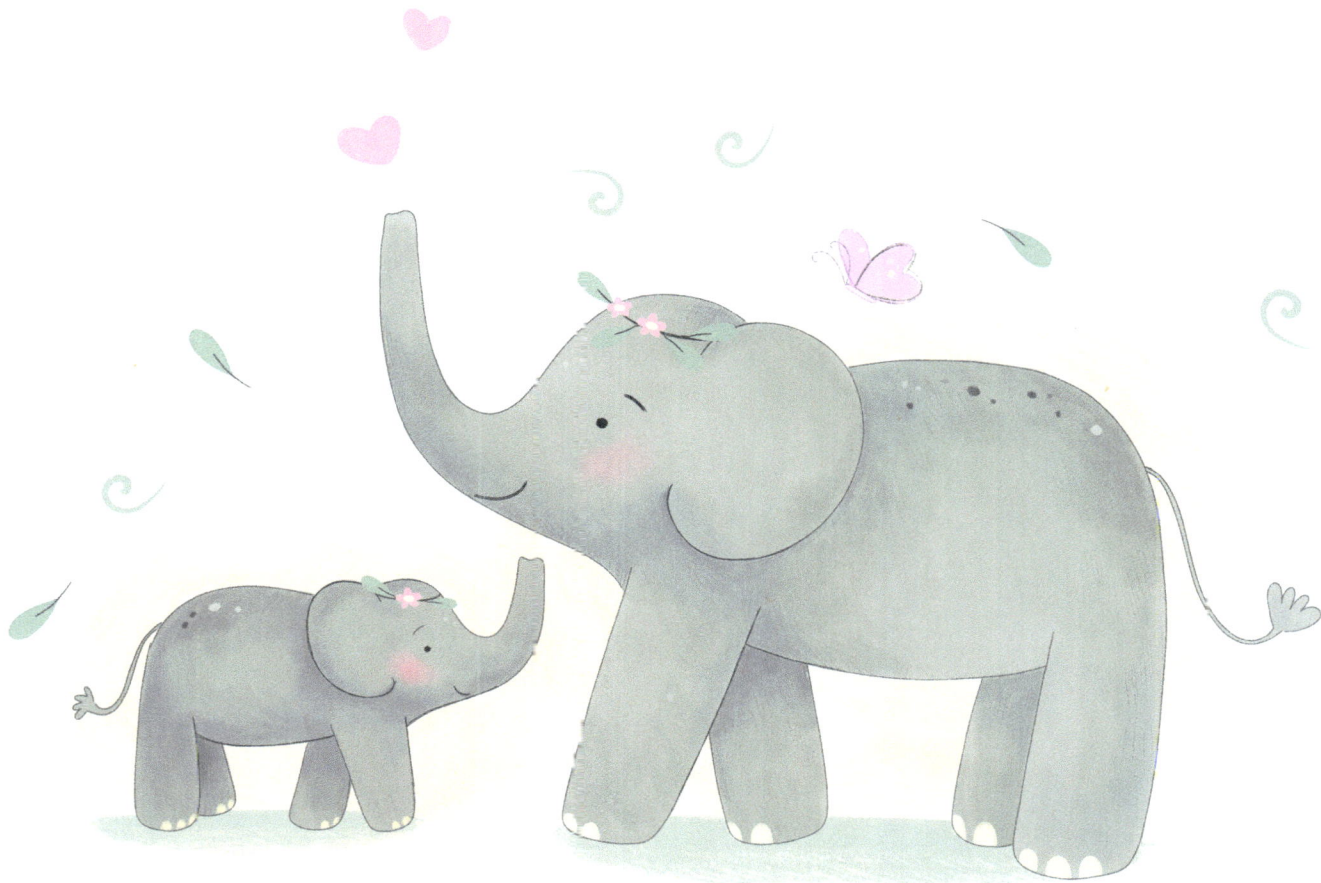

Elephant Mumma,

from the moment you knew I was here

we have been connected.

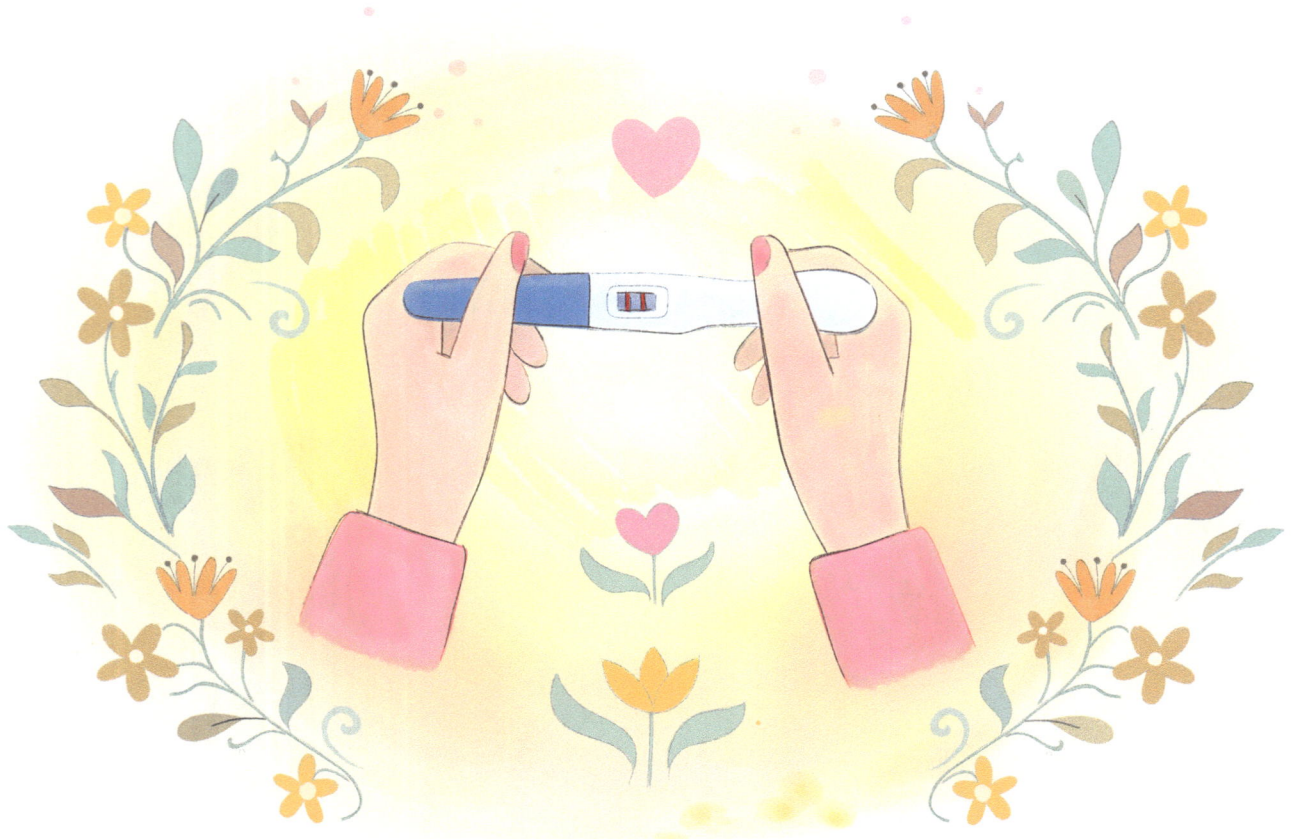

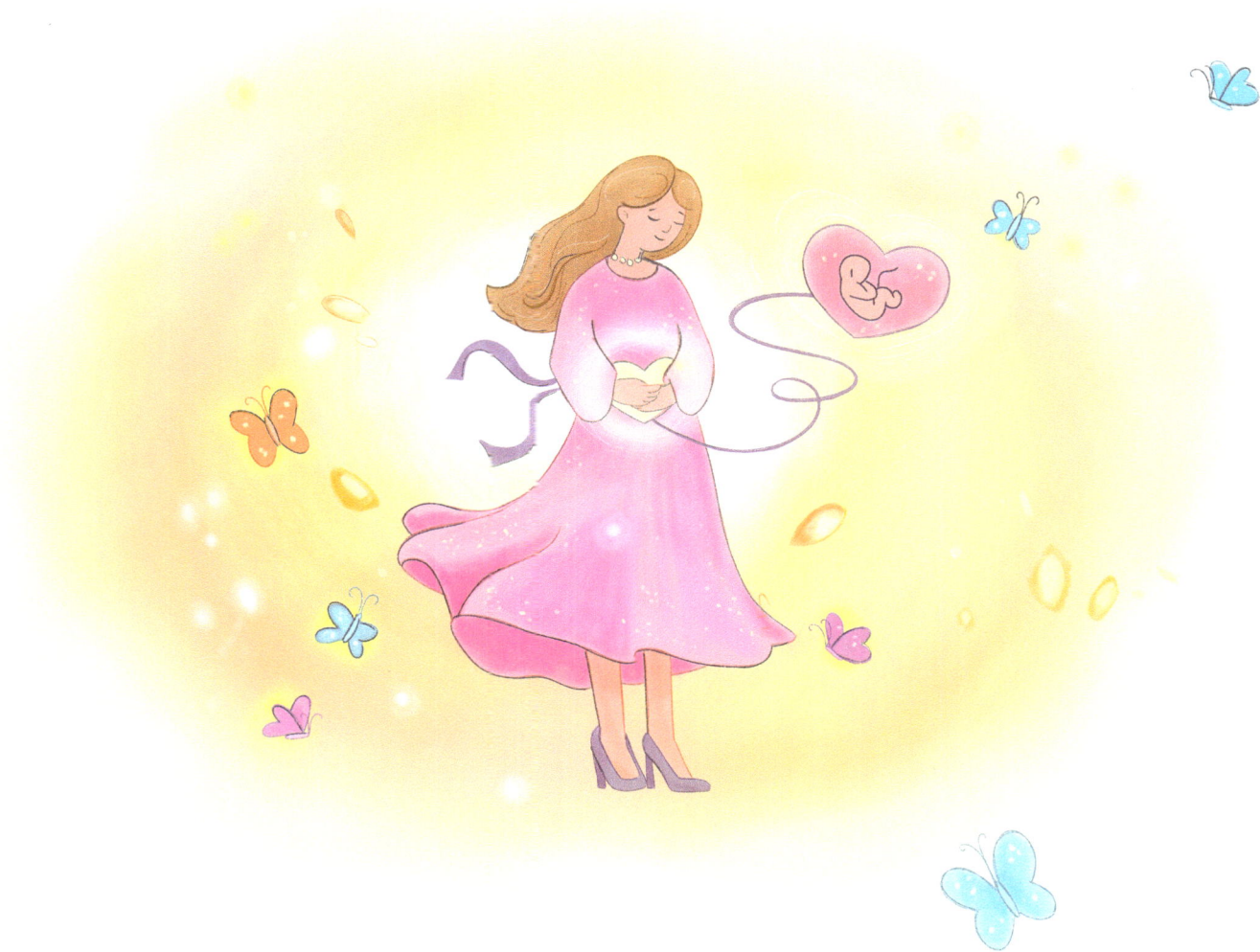

This connection
changes your body and mind,
and grows my body and mind.

Elephant Mumma,
when you think of me,
imagine that with every thought,
my mind is getting to know your mind.

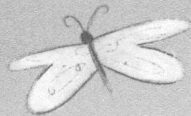

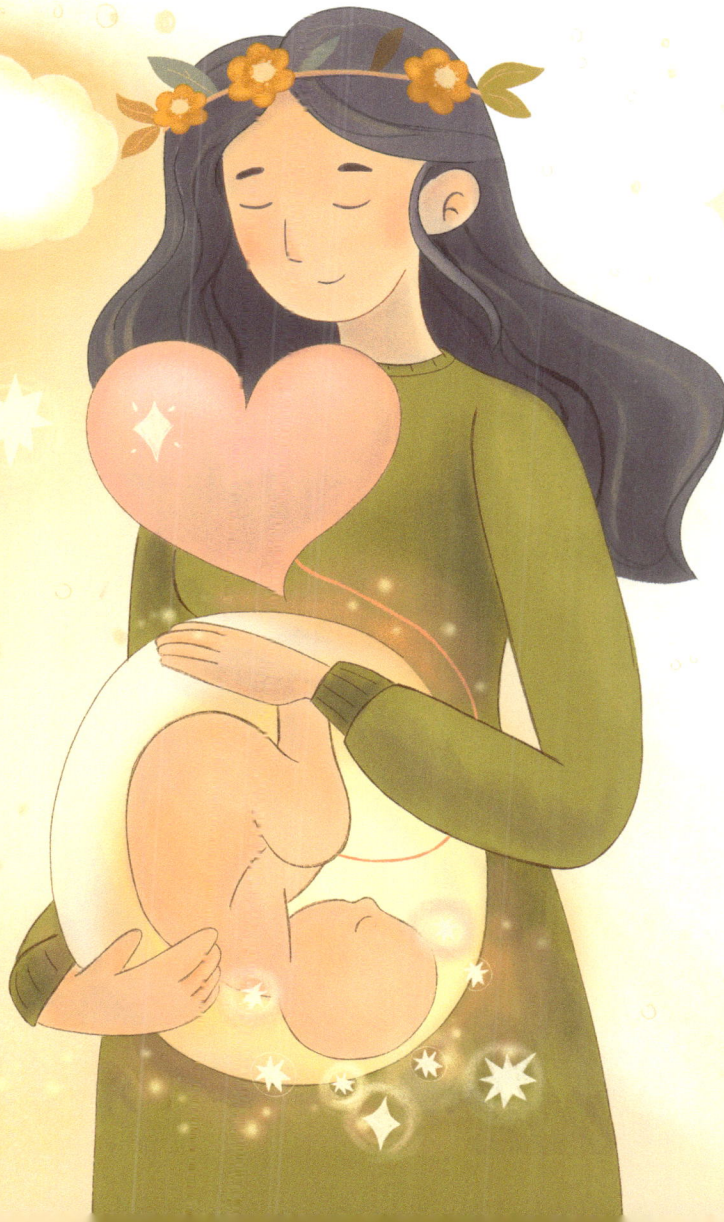

Our minds are like two galaxies,

when you think of me, my stars sparkle.

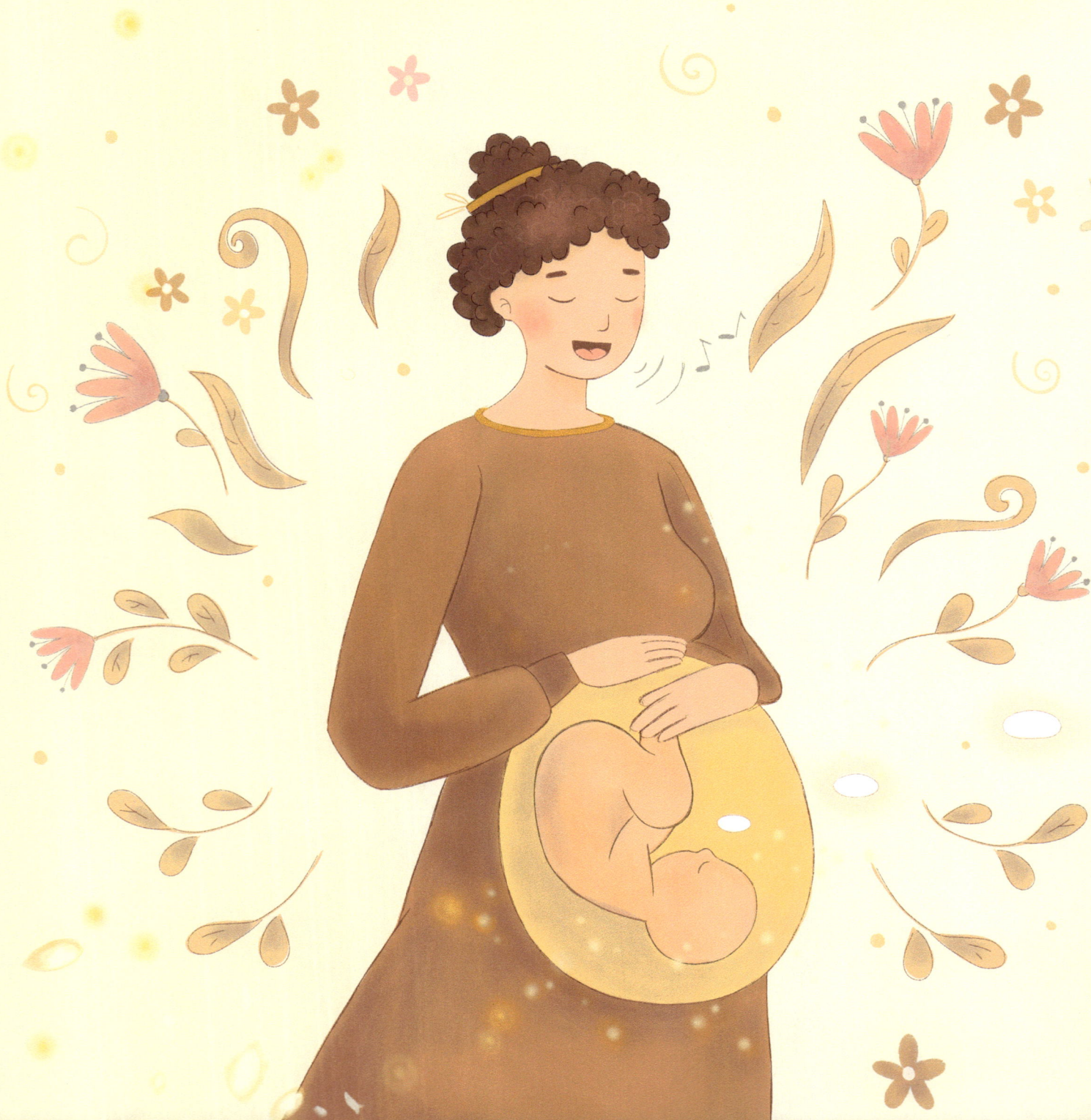

Elephant Mumma,

when you talk to me,

with every sound,

I start to learn your voice.

The soft, kind voices

that I hear are my favourites!

Elephant Mumma,

when you dream about our life together,

I grow even more ready to meet you.

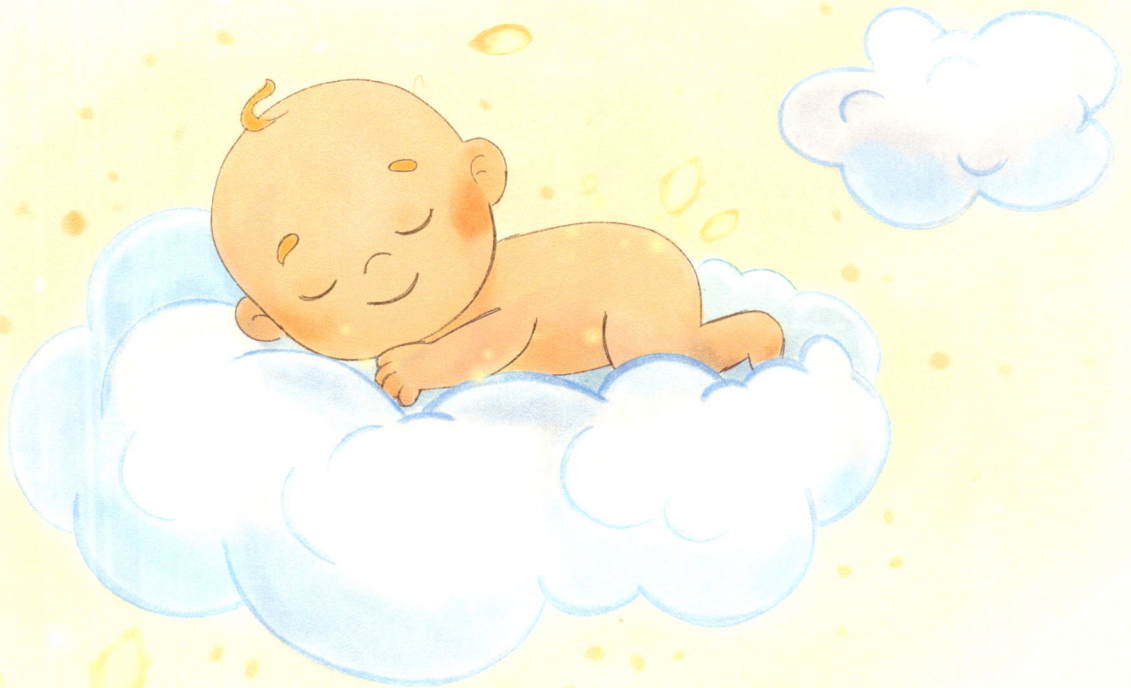

Let your mind wander

towards our future together.

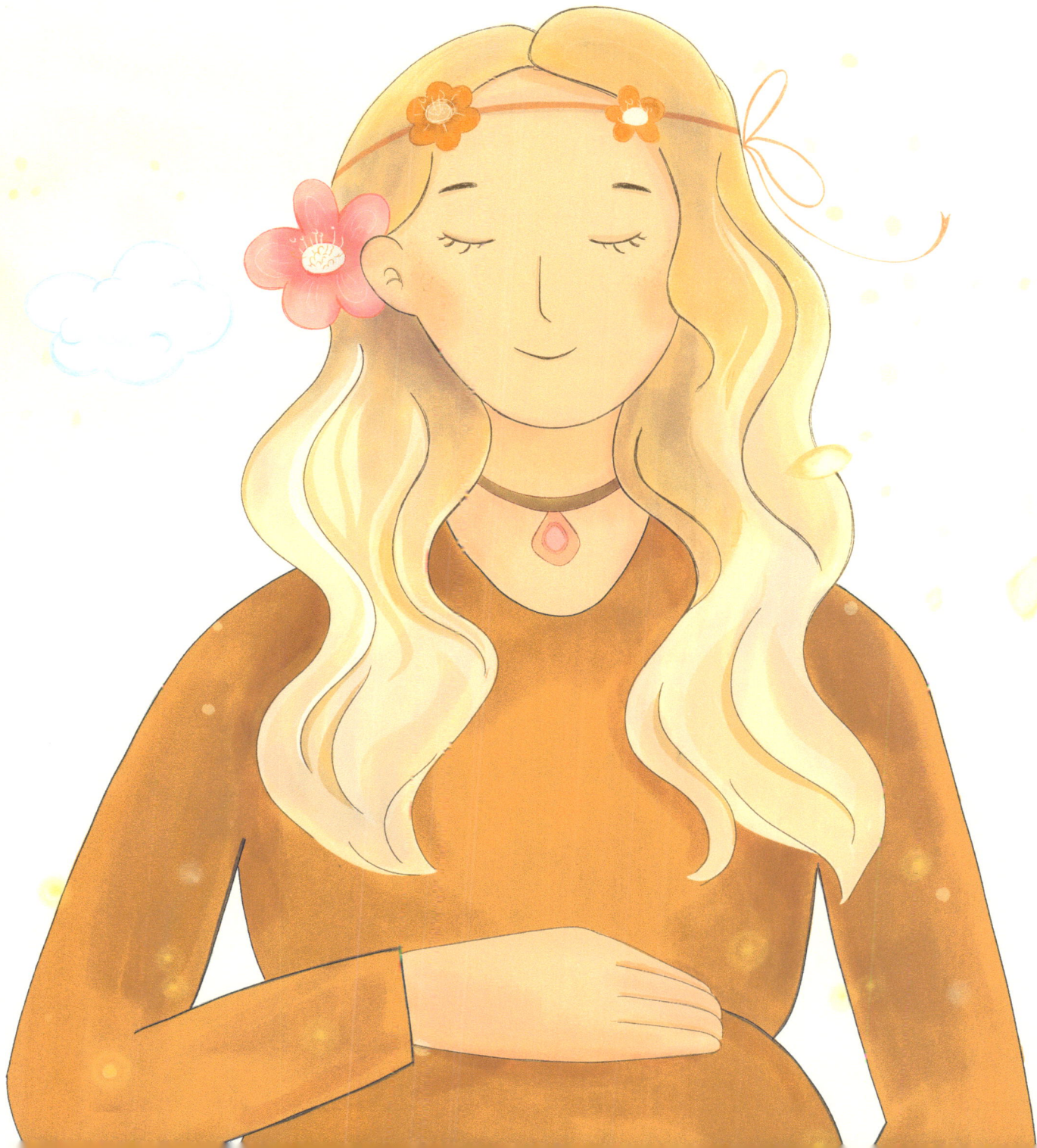

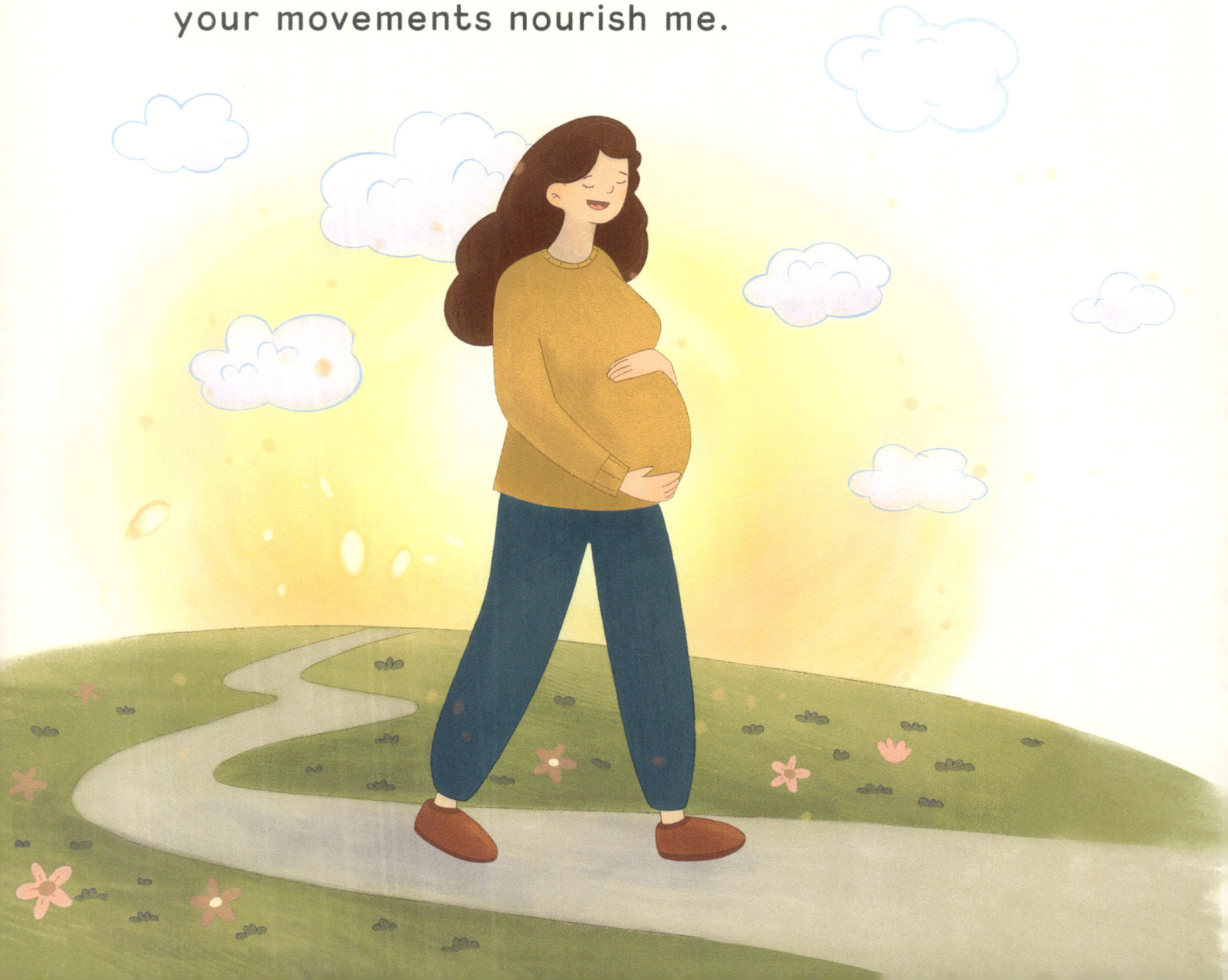

Elephant Mumma,

I like the rhythm of your footsteps,

your movements nourish me.

Take me for a walk, or dance with me!

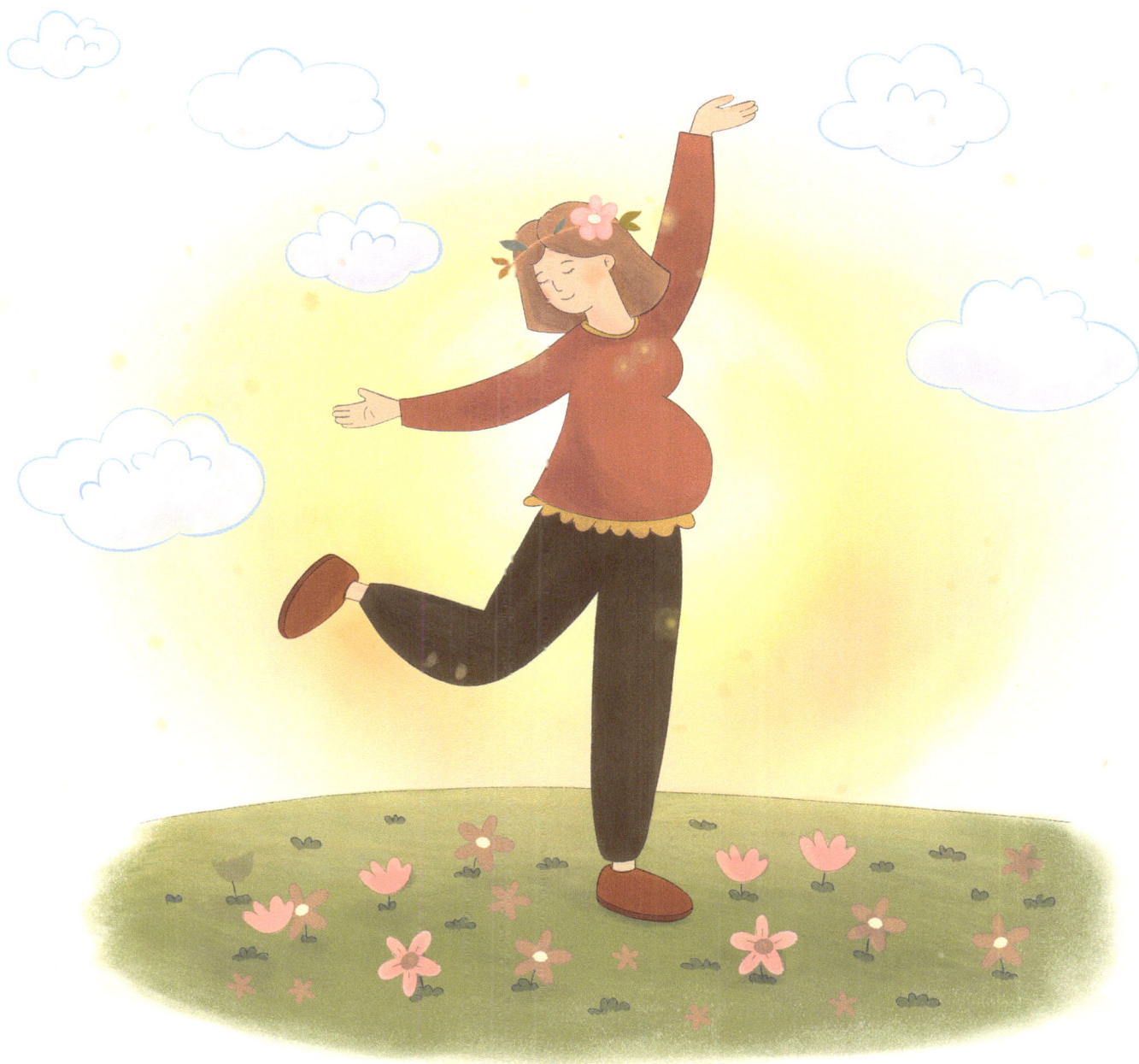

Elephant Mumma, I also like it when we swim.

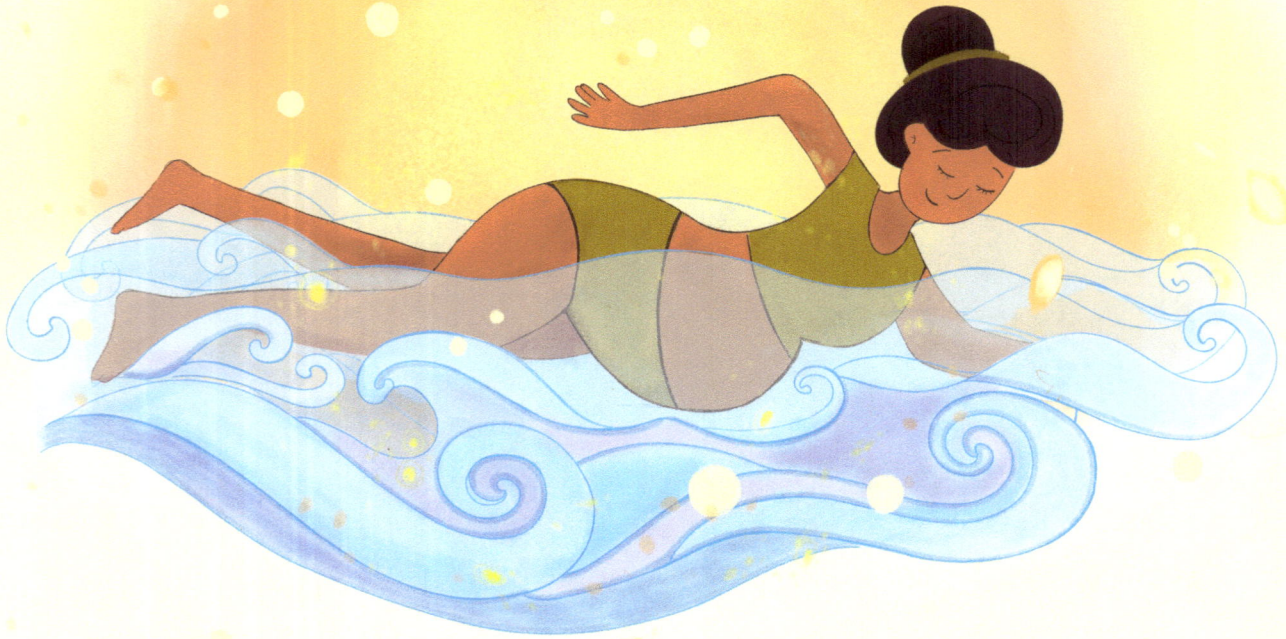

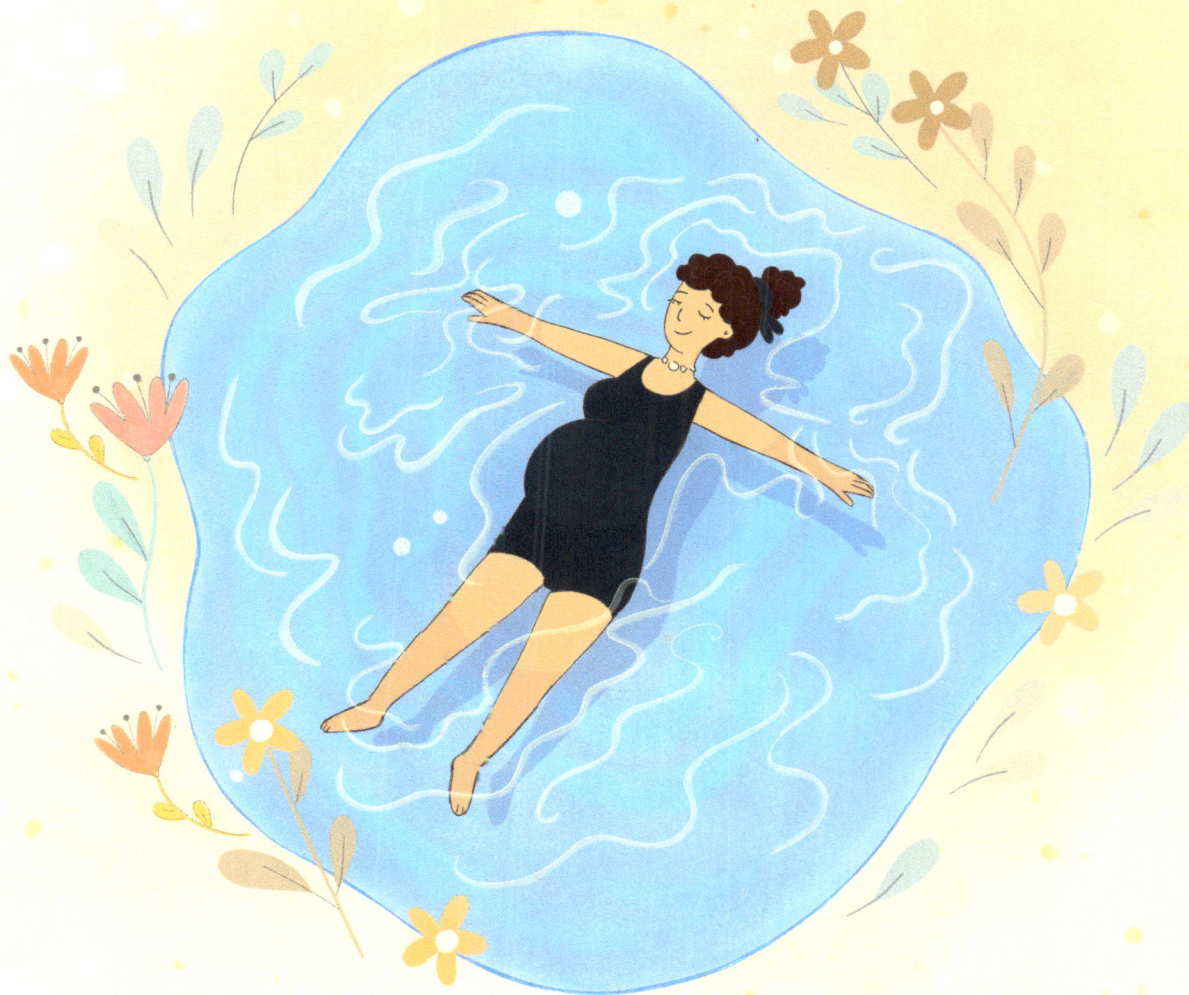

Float with me as I float within you!

Elephant Mumma,
when you breathe in a gentle rhythm,
it soothes me.

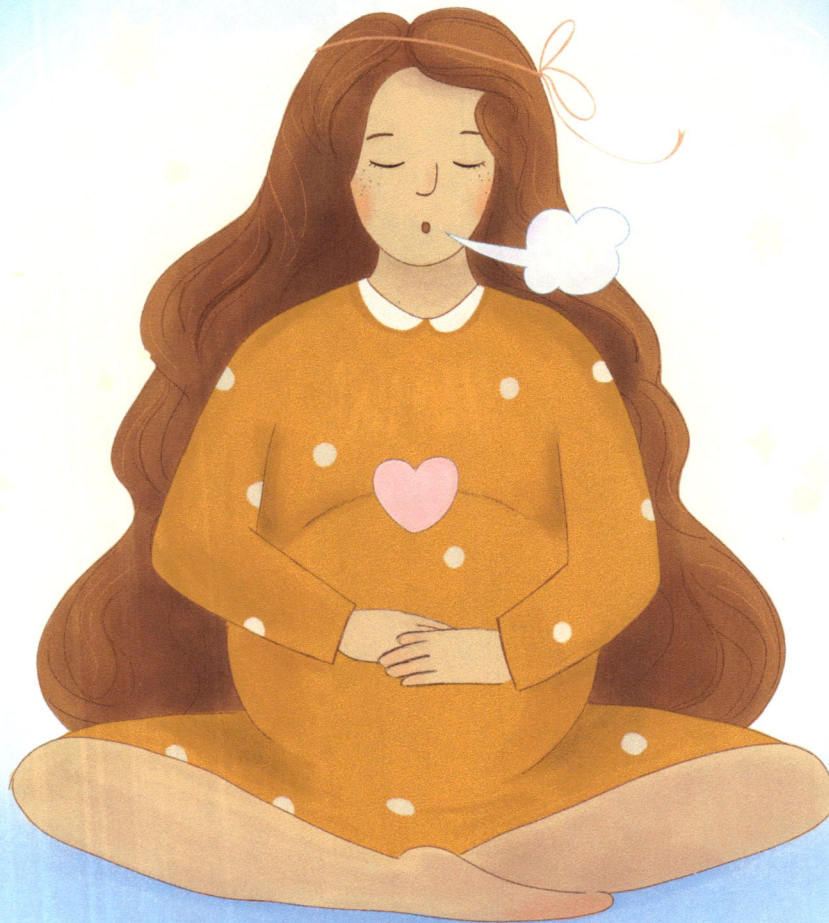

As you breathe in,

trace your finger around the infinity symbol,

and again as you breathe out.

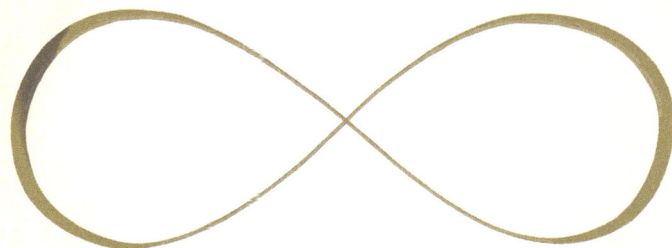

You are breathing for me!

Elephant Mumma,
your heartbeat will be the
first musical rhythm that I hear,
it will always comfort me.

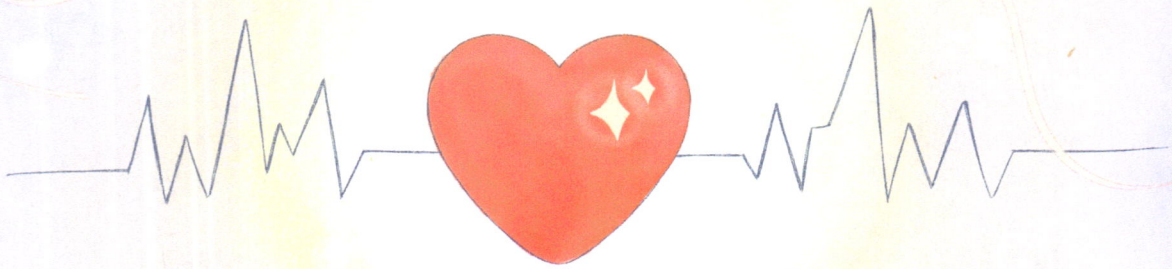

Listen to music with me,
play me your favourite songs,
they might become mine too.

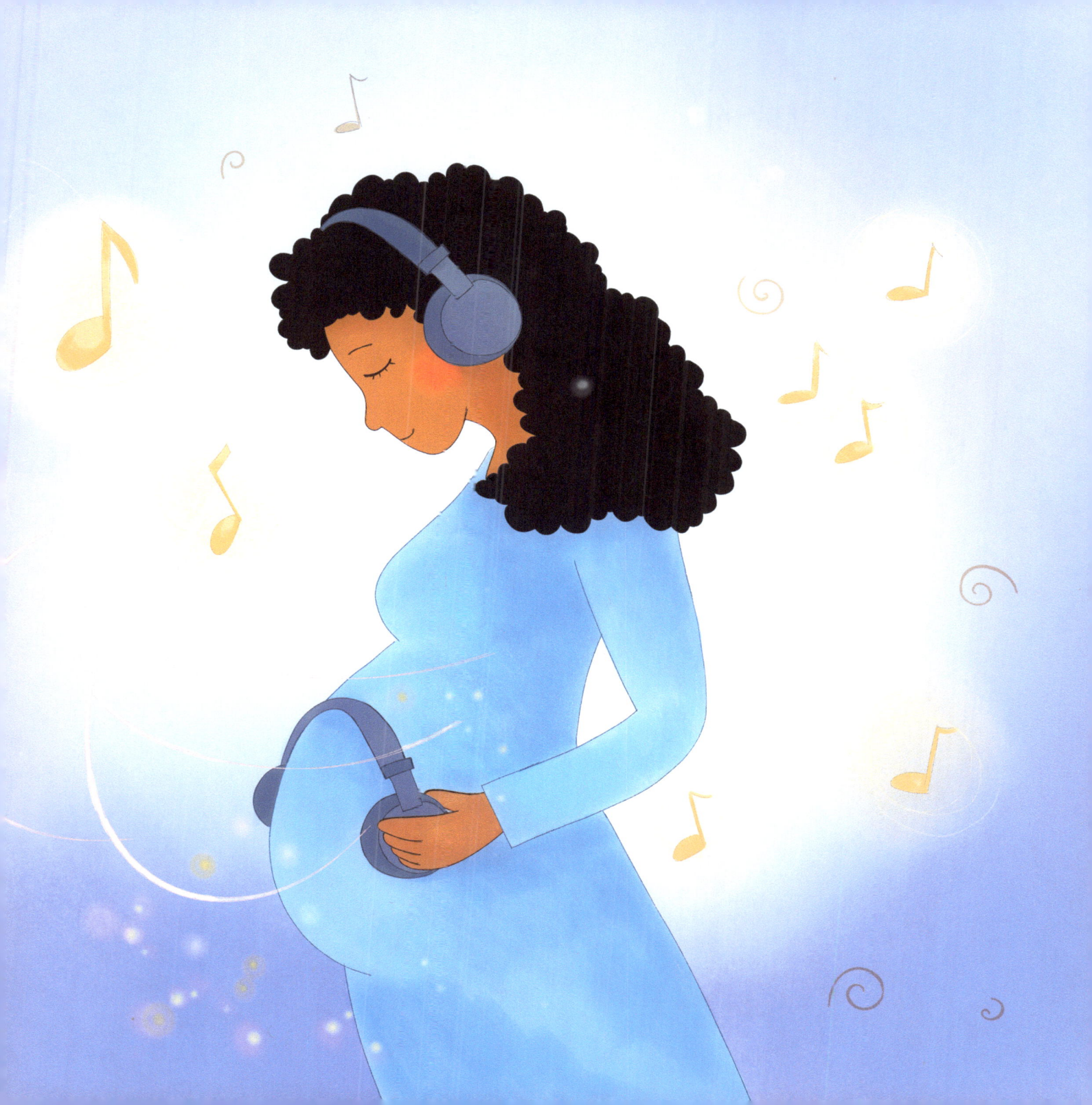

Elephant Mumma,
let your mind wander
back to when you
were a child...

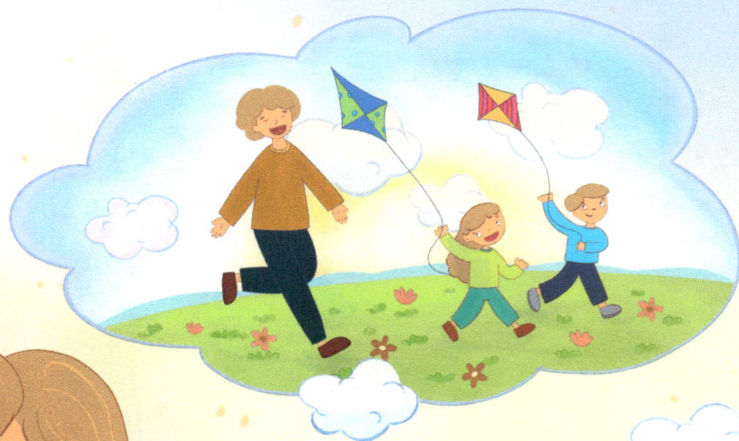

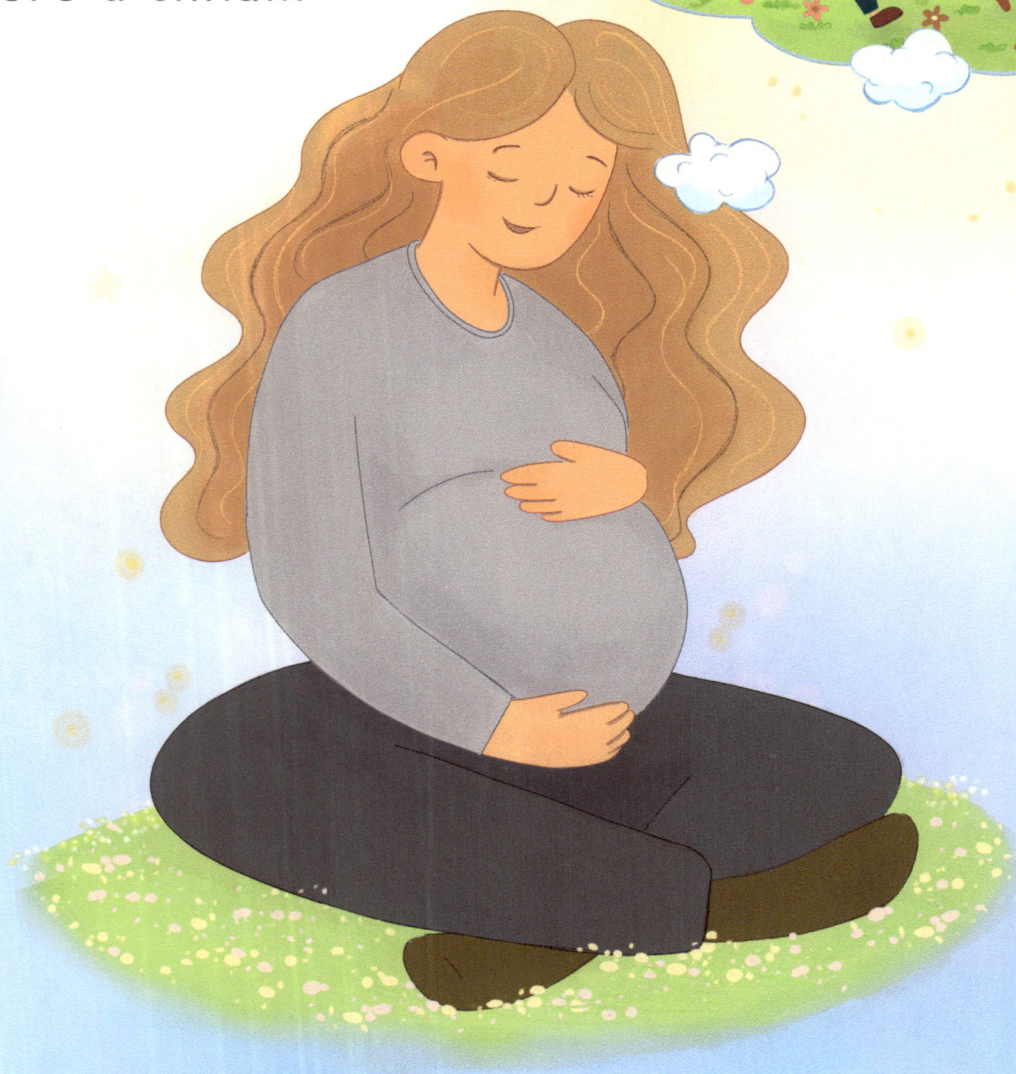

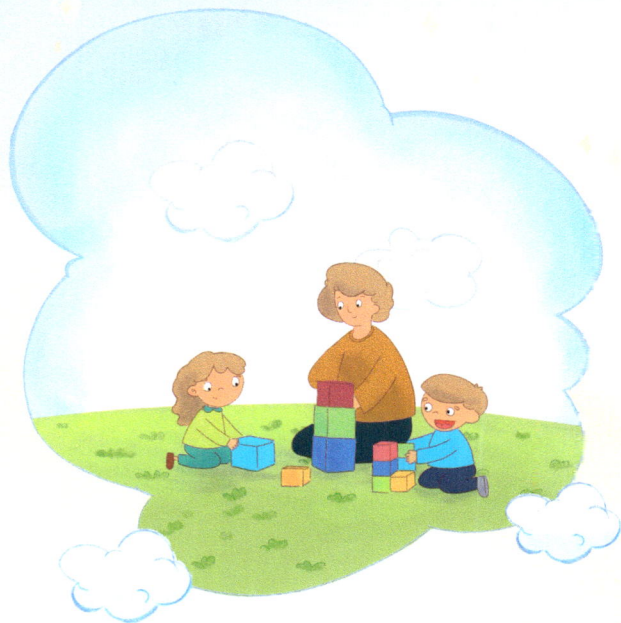

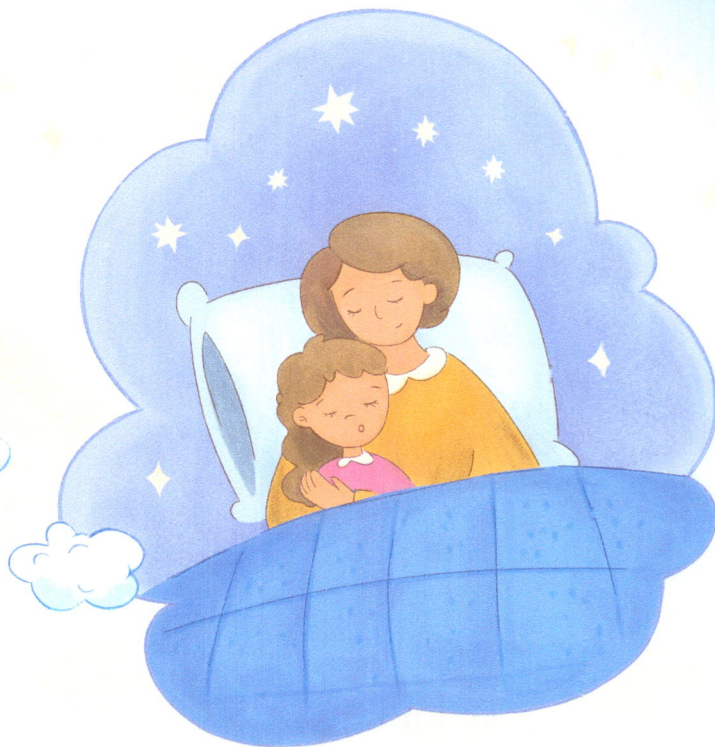

Thinking about your childhood,
the important people and the ways you liked
to play can prepare you to spend time with me!

Elephant Mumma,

if you know any other

Elephant babies or small children,

take me to spend time with them.

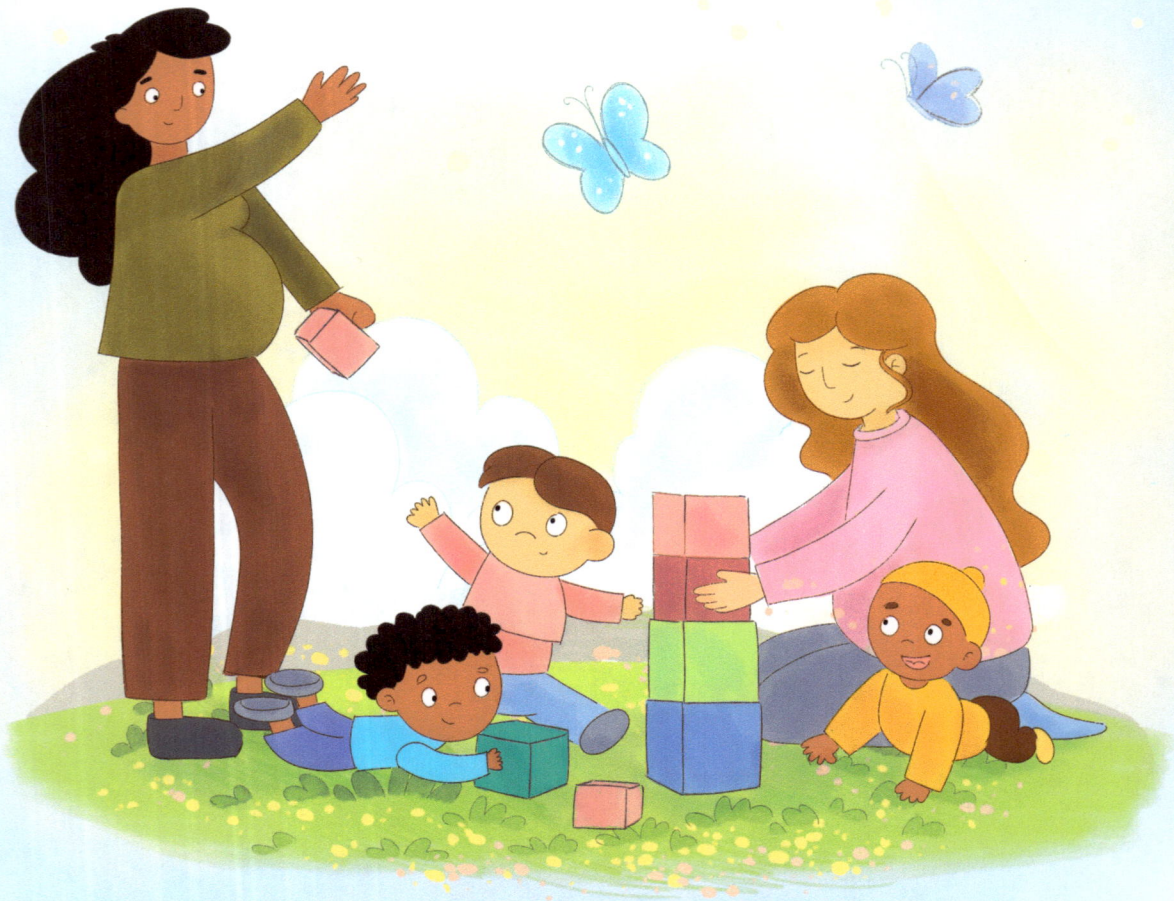

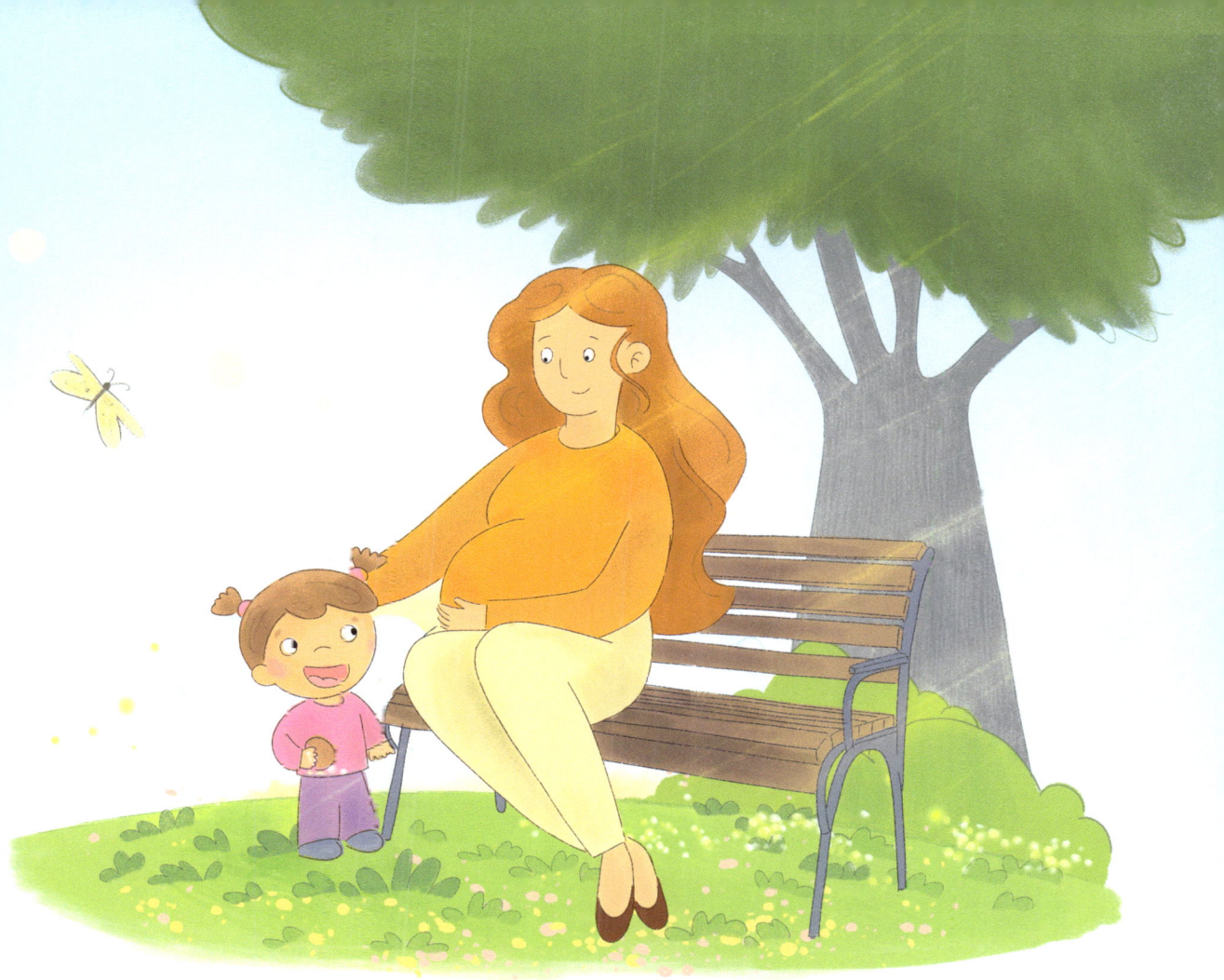

I will enjoy hearing all of the playful noises!
When you watch them play, think about what
they might be feeling, thinking or needing...
this can be good practice for playing with me!

Elephant Mumma,
I love it when you read to me,
I get to hear your heartbeat,
your voice, and I get to know
the rhythm of the books.

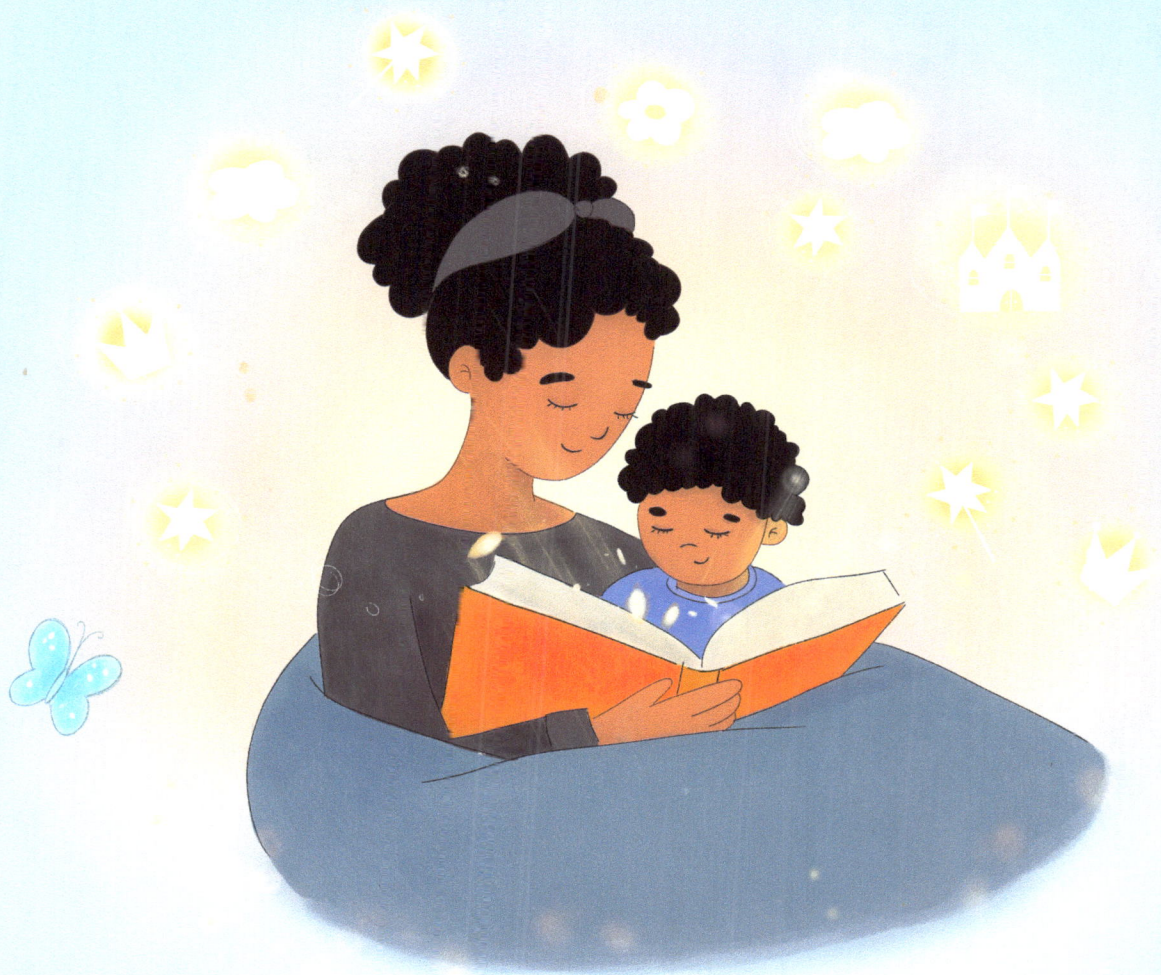

Read this book and other children's books to me as often as you can, they might become the ones we like to read together.

Thank you for reading this
book to me Elephant Mumma!
Give yourself a pat on the back,
a 'woo hoo' or a 'yeehaa!'

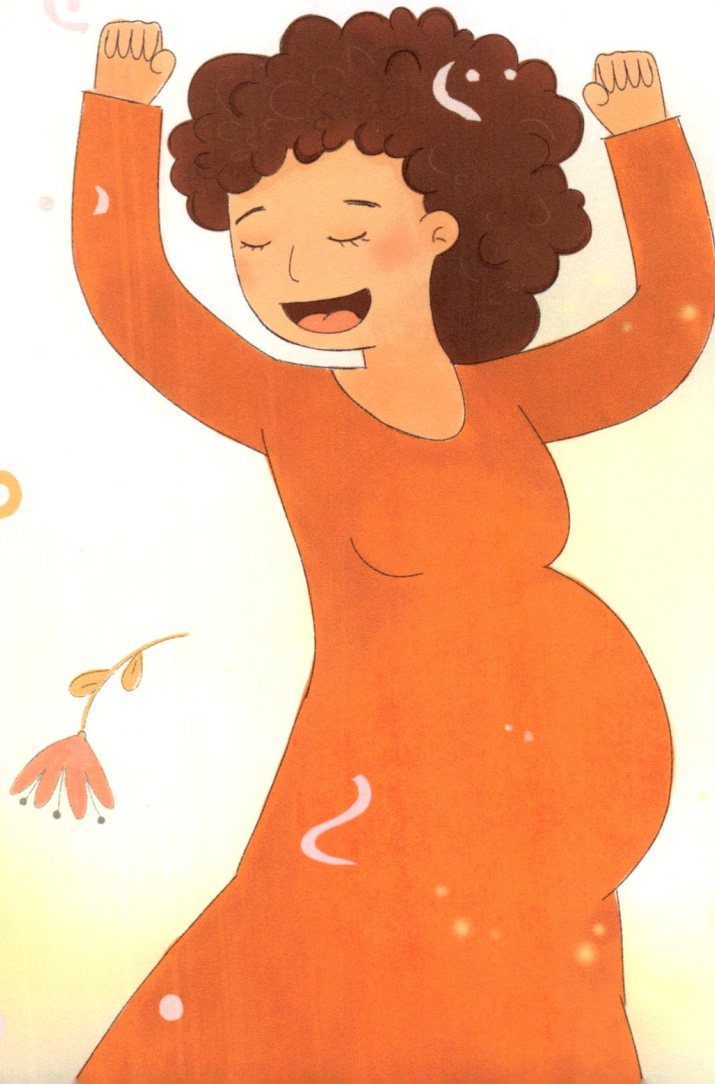

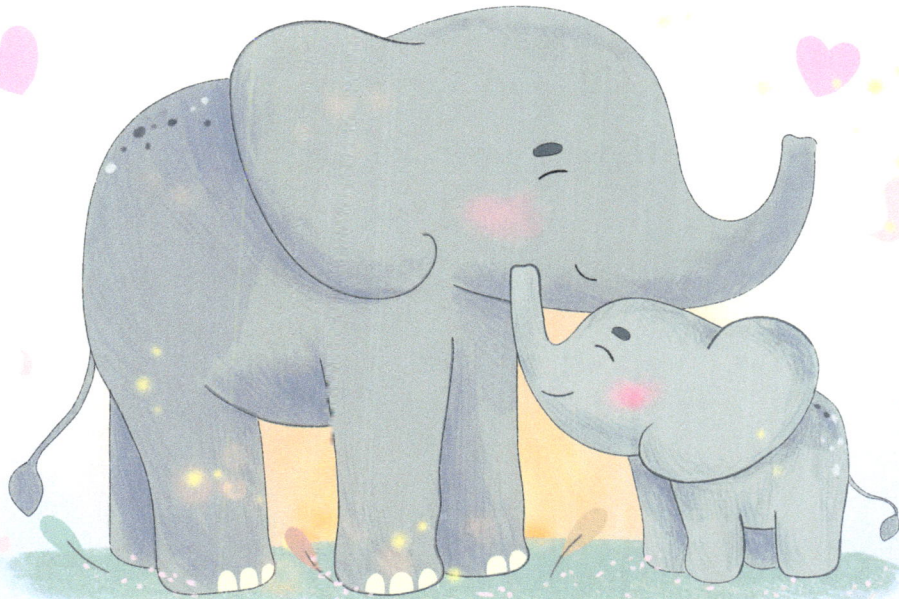

The more you try the things in this book, the bigger and stronger your Elephant heart becomes, and the more my Elephant heart loves you.

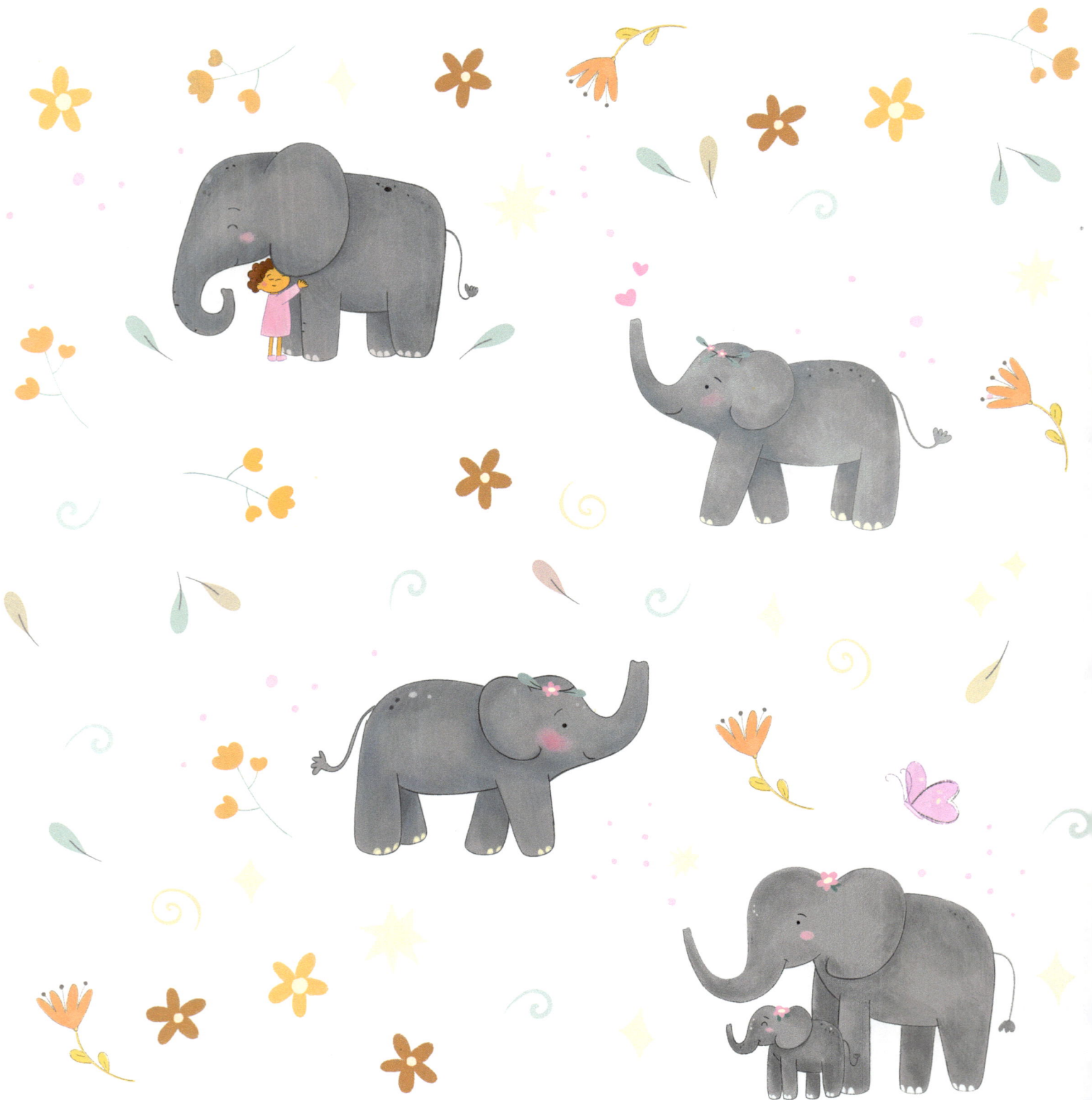

www.ingramcontent.com/pod-product-compliance
Lightning Source LLC
Chambersburg PA
CBHW061136030426
42334CB00003B/66